CARING FOR OTHERS
AMID COVID-19

CARING FOR OTHERS AMID COVID-19

Recruitment and Retention
in Long Term Care

Joseph King Jr.

To order additional copies of this book, contact:
Xlibris
844-714-8691
www.Xlibris.com
Orders@Xlibris.com
825980

This publication is dedicated
to
Joyce Renee King
(In Memoriam)

CONTENTS

ACKNOWLEDGEMENT

I would like to acknowledge the inspiration of Mr. & Mrs. Joseph and Jessie King Sr. (In Memoriam) and family for strong support and encouragement. The participants in this study.

Jay Johnson
Kristall Johnson
Joanne Wilson
Joyce Acklen
Shelley Lee
Corey Boone
&
Rev. D. L. Motley, Jr
Rev. A. A. W. Motley
Rev. D. C. Devonshire

And others were instrumental in providing real world experiences that bring the issues to life. Above all I thank the Almighty for refuge and strength. May God bless us all.

46 Psalm (KJV)

CHAPTER 1

[1] Problem

Caregiver recruitment and caregiver retention all begin by sustaining standards of care, cost structure and customer value. Business model development, job and customer satisfaction are essential in achieving the mission, vision and values of the organization.

Background

Since March 2020 the public at large has become aware of Covid-19. While caring for others was being written, Covid-19 came upon the United States and the world as a global Pandemic. The heroes have been identified as essential personnel. All of the healthcare personnel have been at risk for the own health as well as their family members and friends.

At the time of this writing the death rate has risen to over 850k. (Centers for Disease Control and Prevention (CDC). The recruitment and retention of all long term care industry personnel is critical. Later in the writing pay and benefits to include Personnel Protection Equipment (PPE) will be discussed. A serious incident in New York State affected the long term care industry in a big way. The Governor of New York placed Covid-19 patients in several Skilled Nursing

Facility's (SNF)'s and caused risk to SNF personnel in addition to the demise of numerous patients, despite Federal intervention and support in the form of the hospital ship Comfort and the hospital built in the Jacob Javits Center.

Health Care Workers and Covid-19/CDC

The population of residents in Nursing homes (Skilled Nursing Facilities) (SNF) are affected a big way and are at more risk to Covid-19. Also healthcare workers are at risk due to isolation in the facility and due to residents with Covid-19. The CDC states that SNF's should "assign at least one individual with training in infection prevention and control program is critical to protect both residents and healthcare personnel (HCP)". Further SNF Management must have policies and procedures as well as monitor and audit practices. This practice should be aided by testing, of residents and HCP.

The Infection Control Assessment and Response (ICAR) tool is recommended by the CDC to assess the following

- Keeping Covid-19 out of the facility
- Identify infections as early as possible
- Preventing spread of Covid-19 in the facility
- Assessing and optimizing Personal Protective Equipment (PPE) supplies
- Identifying and managing severe illness in residents with Covid-19

The following areas are addressed in the ICAR tool.

- Visitor restriction
- Education, monitoring, and screening of healthcare personnel (HCP)
- Education, monitoring of residents
- Ensuring availability of PPE and other supplies

- Ensuring adherence to recommended infection prevention and control (IPC) practices.
- Communicating with the health department and other healthcare facilities

The Department of Health and Human Services (HHS) developed and administers the ICAR's for the CDC to combat Covid-19. The development of the aforementioned tool has been developed and deployed at great expense, however the HCP personnel that use and comply with the tool do their jobs everyday at risk to themselves and their families.

Another tool which the CDC uses is the Long-Term Care (LTC) Respiratory Surveillance list this list was developed during March 2020, is designed for HCP and residents, it addresses

- Case Demographics
- Case location
- Signs and symptoms
- Diagnosis
  - type of specimen
  - data collection
  - type of test ordered
  - pathogen detected
- Outcome during outbreak https:/www.cdc.gov/longtermcare/training.html
- Outbreak summary

The aforementioned tools depict a great deal of the response to Covid-19 in SNF's, again the workers' (HCP) compensation has not improved before, and during this pandemic. Today, there are not any role models to benchmark against as it relates to pay, benefits and compensation.

The Maclom Baldrige National Quality Award has a framework that can and is used to identify role model organizations and does a good job of it, however none of the role model healthcare/long term care organizations reveal and document significant pay and compensation strategies for improving pay, benefits and compensation. In Baldrige Examiner speak, this is an Opportunity For Improvement "OFI".

Currently the CDC indicates that healthcare is the fastest growing sector of the US economy. This sector employees over 18 million people. Workers in this industry are not only at risk due to Covid-19. Exposures to blood contamination, inadvertent needle pricks, muscle strains, and lifting injuries are also problematic. I must make a distinction between workers' compensation insurance and pay and benefits. The focus of this writing is on pay and benefits primarily and workers compensation insurance secondarily. Workers compensation insurance not only covers medical expenses and lost wages, but employees can also receive benefits such as mileage, vocational rehabilitation and Activities for Daily Living (ADL) that come as a result of all accident or incident.

Covid-19 Pay, Benefits and Injuries

In addition to Covid-19 issues, the long term care industry employees face some of the highest rates of on the job injuries across all industries to include construction, nursing and manufacturing. Most of the injuries of employees are musculoskeletal.

Data from the Bureau of Labor Statistics, indicate that employees working at nursing homes and long term care facilities experience rates of injury that are seven times higher than the average across all industries. Most the injuries are related to moving, transporting and repositioning patients https://pmcinsurance.com/reducing-workers-compensation-claims-at-long-term-care-facilities.

This information reveals that long term care employees, face danger on a daily basis, without being impacted by Covid-19. These impacts make it difficult to recruit and retain employees that "care for others".

Uncovering the Devaluation of Nursing Home Staff during Covid-19

"Currently a significant portion of deaths are attributed to persons living in nursing homes ranging from 42% to 57% in European countries reporting data, to as high as 82% in several US states and in Canada. However, there is a concern that many countries are not including nursing home deaths in the death toll."

Many experts predict and believe nursing home staff who will die from Covid-19 are adjunct nursing home staff. (Editorial JAMDA 21 (2020) 967-965) www.jamda.com

Understaffing has been a chronic challenge globally in the Long Term Care (LTC) industry. Providing care makes LTC leadership more challenging. Understaffing makes following Covid protocols more difficult. This can impact behaviors in residents with dementia who may not understand or follow the procedures. "Precarious working conditions, characterized by part-time employment, heavy workloads, primitive measures related to sick time, low wages, and an obligation to work when sick contribute to a global staffing crises in nursing homes." IBID(1).

Furthermore, "nursing homes are working under capacity as staff have tested positive for Covid-19 symptoms. At the same time, some countries report significant rates of staff absenteeism or abandonment of their work because of fear of getting the virus or transmitting it to love ones. This fear is not unfounded, many staff providing the most hands on, direct care in nursing homes (e.g. bathing, assisting with meals) are women, who have doubled or triple caregiving responsibilities with a low socioeconomic status that cannot risk income loss regardless of working conditions, and are at high risk for poor health outcomes if infected". IBID(2)

Nursing home healthcare has always been marginalized in favor of acutcare healthcare facilities (hospitals). The nursing home health care worker has been the "second string". An example from another industry shows the point of view.

US Army

The US Army has three major components.

1. Active Army (Regular Army)
2. Army National Guard
3. Army Reserve

Warfighters (combatants) are housed primarily in the Active Army. Army National Guards men and women are affiliated and assigned to states, but can be mobilized in time of war. Army Reservists are engaged in combat service, and combat service support. Yet vital to the total force, Army reservists have been historically undervalued and although they are also mobilized in time war, they are still considered the second string. Understanding that Reserve Commanders have been elevated in rank and responsibility, the stigma of being "less than" the others still lingers despite the importance of the mission and mission needs. As we labeled both groups "our heroes", the pay and prestige yet remains in the primary care group in healthcare and in the Active Army. Stigma remains when a value propositive is not enacted, followed by equality of opportunity from a "fundamental fairness" prospective.

"We as a global society, have failed our nursing home community residents, relatives, and staff. Given that this pandemic has publicly revealed and aggravated the long standing old age precarious working conditions in nursing homes, it can be reasonably expected that future recruitment of staff will be a greater challenge." IBID (4):

A. Who are the caregivers in long-term healthcare?

The caregivers are varied. Informally, they may be aunt, uncle, sister, brother or any family member. Sometimes they are adult children or a spouse, male or female. Again they are varied and as we approach 2030, these caregivers mentioned may assume a greater role as homecare is becoming a preferred way of spending time in home care instead of in a facility. Much is written about the formal caregivers in a skill nursing facility (SNF,) assisted living (AL) or special long-term care facility (LTCF). Caregiver support is critical as the relationship with the resident, family member or spouse is given more attention as well as concern. Different types of client's are also residing in SNFs.

[2] The research on retention

Generally focuses on administrators, nurses, social workers, medical directors, consultants, support pharmacists and therapists. "Some research, although still very little, could be found in the literature about job satisfaction among professional long-term care staff and factors influencing their intention to stay in or leave their positions." 1. Also, there is a paucity of information on non-professional caregivers which were previously mentioned.

As most organization's focus on the customer (resident) for mission effectiveness and customer value, oftentimes the caregiver is an "internal customer" and their work/life balance to include "job satisfaction" is equally important. The research is still lacking as it addresses the caregiver professional or non-professional staff.

[3] Nursing facility administrators have challenges with retention.

- Independent facilities had higher retention rates than multi-facility chains
- Facility size is important in retention
- Administrator commitment has a positive effect on retention

C Singh and Schwab (1998)

The basic industry by these writers state that job satisfaction and organizational commitment are significant in retaining administrators.

Also, nurses have challenges with retention:

- Most research addresses the direct service worker, the certified nursing assistant (CNA) as it should however, the registered nurse (RN,) or Director of Nursing (DON) are caregivers as well.

Castle and Englserg (2006)

- discovered turnover rates at 35.8%. Generally these numbers are combined (RN plus LPN)

[4] "Lower CNA staffing levels, however, as well as lower nursing home quality, for profit facility ownership status and greater bed size were associated with higher combined nursing turnover." 2.

Social workers are also in need of retention efforts to improve the workplace environment. Again, a paucity of research addresses this concern. A major study by Whiteaker, Wermeuller and Clark, 2006, P29 addresses the need for more action to improve the practice environment, which addresses, case load, higher salary, job stress and family concerns.

"In addition those with a master's degree in social work serving older clients earn the highest salary in private practice hospitals and the lowest in nursing homes." Whitaker T, Weisminer T. and Clark (2006) 3.

[5] Medical Directors, consultant pharmacists and therapists also have challenges however; the lack of research is obvious. Discussions about the field speak to the need for quality, performance effectiveness and improvement of the environment. The lack of research signals a need for research to address the needs of all employees who work in the long-term care industry.

B. Trends and Challenges

As growing needs for trend data that tracks supply and demand for potential shortages is needed. The Baby Boomer generation as it grows requires long-term care services.

- Further studies should address turnover and vacancy rates to determine the impact.
- The characteristics of the long-term care work force, particularly needs assessment of non-professional caregivers.
- [6] The impact of wage and recruitment and retention in long term care.
- Focuses on quality outcomes and working conditions.
- The relationship between job satisfaction and long-term care quality is significant. (IFAS) January 2007)

Challenges

- Wage and benefit studies are needed to address the impact on recruitment and retention efforts for direct care personnel, CNA's and LPN's.
- Education and training reforms to evaluate costs recruitment, retention, job satisfaction and quality of care.
- Organizational and staffing innovations to assign work tasks, such as selecting, assigning [7] and supervising staff.
- The impact of payments to family (non-professional) caregivers. The impact of payments beyond stipends can assist in reducing the demand for care and increase recruitment and retention.

While the government and the private sector address these needs along with organizations such as the National Baldrige Quality Award (NBQA) program and the American Health Care Association (AHCA). Additional workshops with facilities can better equip organizations in developing business models and value propositions for customers to address caregiver needs and the overall mission, vision and value of the organization.

CHAPTER 2

[8] Discussion and Interviews

To add realism to the research it is important in the here and now to ask questions of caregivers and their customers to include family members of the client (patient, resident, family member, spouse, etc....) as well as family members as clients. All of the aforementioned clients are all customers to include the caregivers as seen by the SNF.

"Value Proposition Design" by Oscar Walder A. Pignew 4. Bermarda Smith A 2014. P.G. describe the customer profile as having "gains," which describe the outcomes customers want to achieve, benefits they are seeking, "pains" describe the outcomes, risks and obstacles related to customer jobs, and customer jobs describe what customers are trying to get done in their work and in their lives, as expressed in their own words." 4.

[9] In an interview with John/Jane Doe 1

A family member and her daughter taking care of a spouse at home was a deeply stressful endeavor, while support was given by the Veterans Administration Hospital (VA), the task was mentioned as being overwhelming. There was much interaction with the VA administrator, Director of Nursing (DON), social worker, and a host of caregivers assigned to the client by the VA in coordination with the various local health care agencies. John/Jane Doe 1 as a recent retiree and spouse (client) retiree was entering a "new world". While both retirees where government employees and were familiar with bureaucracy, a new bureaucracy emerged. Key in the discussion was that the family member(s) became co-caregivers with the assigned personnel from the healthcare agency (HCA) and the VA.

Many customer pains where experienced by John/Jane Doe 1 to include the following:

[10] Pains

- inconsistent care by the caregivers assigned to the household to include, caregivers working multiple jobs and coming to the home unprepared (e.g. doing college homework or social media activities)
- HCA states a lack of caregivers are available to cover needed times of care
- lack of social work support for family caregivers (e.g. counseling, assistance while serving 24 hour coverage in the home)
- lack of coordination between VA administration and HCA personnel to assist family customers

*An Army of caregivers coming and going, and having no relationship with the family or client."

[11]

- A need and request for Congressional involvement (congressional inquiry) to assist in remedying issues with VA personnel to include the administration regarding issues dealing with caregivers, family member support, social work support and VA benefits for the services member client.

Gains:

- effective congressional support from the State/Congressional Representative and US Senator
- Learning the process and making it work to help others.
- Understanding assigned caregiver pains e.g. the need to work, several jobs due to pay and benefits.
- **[12]** Understanding the issues in Health Care Agency (HCA) administration and the need for more caregivers and proper scheduling of caregivers.
- The primary gain is in making the system work to receive concrete benefits for the client, but not for family member caregivers.

As discussed with John/Jane Doe 1 this issue of support for family member caregivers is still left open, in that the loss of a loved one is enough, however, the lingering needs of the family member caregiver was not addressed.

[13] In an interview with John/Jane Doe 2

A twenty-five (25) plus year caregiver who has worked for many health care agencies (HCA) and whose career has resulted in working for families providing direct care the experience has distinct similarities and slight differences.

Pains

- Gross inconsistencies in salary and benefits over the twenty-five-year period.
- The need to take on additional jobs (e.g. bath care, multiple clients.)
- The need to work for multiple (HCA) agencies at the same time.

- Inconsistent salary and benefits, over the time period to include a lack of professional development education.
- A lack of an advocacy group to address, caregiver needs and support.
- No recovery assistance from client loss and coping.
- A lack of supplies. (e.g. soap, gloves, towels.)
- Short staffing, 1 to 15 clients, too many residents to care for at one time.
- A lack of supervising support to include social work personnel and administrator support.
- Highly directive family members in a home environment.

[15] Gains

- Working with clients (life's work) and enjoying the fact that "I can care for others that cannot care for themselves".
- Personalities of clients (seeing them become more independent in rehabilitation cases and gain more confidence.)
- Working with families, friends of family and the clergy.
- Working with other caregivers in a "team work" environment in the SNF as well as in home environment.
- Resolving issues and giving clients a better quality of life and hoping "I will get the same quality of care when I need it."

Interview John/Jane Doe 3

Family Caregiver Supported by Professionals, a daughter providing support to her mother being new to the caregiver role.

GAINS

1. Wisdom transferred thru in depth conversations
2. Evolving friendship
3. Unanswered questions addressed
4. Ability to celebrate the good days

PAINS

1. Realization that death is close
2. Watching physical deterioration
3. Increasing pressure to meet needs
4. Giving up your personal life as you knew it
5. Coping with their diminishing abilities
6. Asking your parents to give up their independence
7. Lack of family participation
8. Knowing that it is the last Thanksgiving, Christmas etc.
9. Aware of calendar and the prognosis date
10. Being afraid of getting the phone call
11. The reality of knowing what's coming
12. Death

Interview with John/Jane Doe 4

<u>Family Care</u>

Gains:

Family member is with you on a daily basis which gives you the opportunity to take care of them directly and to know their needs are being met all of the time and the quality of care being given

Family member is able to stay in a residence that they are familiar and comfortable with, (knows the lay of the land); have access to their favorite chair or comfortable bed

Family member can continue to be cared for medically by doctors who have previously been monitoring her/his care. Doctors who know her/his medical history and with whom the family member knows and are comfortable with

Family member's personal belongings are not broken, misplaced or stolen as they are not subject to being handled by persons who are not conscientious, caring or honest

Family member is not subject to the illness or uncontrollable behavior of other people

Pains:

Caregiver's life is consumed with providing care; you neglect yourself (wants and needs)

Caregiver feels helpless and guilty when the family member they are caring for gets sicker because the caregiver thinks they should have done something different or better; that the care they gave was not good enough

Having to keep the family member in a residence that now presents safety hazards to the family member due to her/his mental or physical health because the caregiver is unable to correct or change conditions due to lack of funds to make the necessary changes or repairs or feeling angry and/or resentful because of having to use funds to make the home safe for the family member when the caregiver really cannot afford to do so

Not knowing or being able to directly provide the type of medical treatment needed in the event an emergency situation occurs with the family member; not having medical personnel readily available to handle an emergency or crisis situation

Caregiver feeling resentful or angry at siblings or other family members because of the caregiver's perception of their lack of help and support

Caregiver feeling overwhelmed but afraid or resistant to ask for help for fear of looking incapable or not in control

Nursing Home Care

Knowledgeable health care staff are at the facility 24hrs. a day in order to address the daily needs of the family member and in the event of an emergency health care issues with the family member

Facility designed to safely house the family member

Family caregiver no longer needs to neglect her/his physical, mental and emotional health needs; able to take time for self (something as simple as getting a good night sleep)

There is always someone available to watch the family member so they don't have to be taken out in inclement/bad weather or left alone

Activities are offered for the residents to keep them busy and entertained

Pains:

Staff not adequately trained to effectively handle the responsibilities associated with their job

The ratio of nursing assistant staff to residents is not sufficient so it limits the timeliness and quality of care given to each residents

Not all staff are conscientious or caring

Due low pay and the demands in caring for the residents there is a constant turnover of staff which results in a lack of consistency in the residents' care

In order to fill the vacancies timely many staff are hired on a per diem basis which results in staff not really getting to know the residents and their needs

Doctors assigned to care for the family member are hired by the nursing home, they don't know the family member's medical history and are not readily available to her/his family; they don't have regular office hours at the nursing home

Family member has to adjust to an unfamiliar setting and be in contact with other residents who may have serious health problems or behavior issues

The family member's personal items are misplaced, lost or stolen

Not all activities offered are relevant for all the residents in the nursing home

The family who identifies the breakdown in the services and/or complains about the quality of care provided by the nursing home and its staff are often seen as problematic or labeled as a troublemaker as opposed to being appreciated for trying help improve the quality of care and services

The family still has to be actively involved in the daily care (including health care) given to the family member even though they are paying a large sum of money for the nursing home staff to do it

[16] Again, as determined from the interviews the discussion highlights that fact that caregiver retention as well as recruitment is becoming critical as we address standards of care and quality of care. Clients to caregiver ratios are of significant value when addressing costs of care, cost structure and revenue streams for administrators, key resources are vital in offering and delivering quality services. "In the for profit environment, profit is determined and calculated by subtracting the total of all costs in the cost structure from the total of all revenue streams" (OscarWaler, Pigneur, Bernarda and Smith. 2014) in the not for profit environment cost structure is yet again significant in the use of tax payer dollars and revenue to support quality long-term care for [17] an ever growing number of Baby Boomer clients as well as rehabilitation care by those that will use SNFs.

CHAPTER 3

Solutions

As we next discuss solutions it is imperative that we understand that policy solutions at the government level with Medicare/Medicaid to assist in recruitment and retention efforts in long term care but, how long will it take and so what? So what are our opportunities for improvement (OFI) how long can we wait on the current condition to exacerbate? What will government policies add to the problem? What can we do here and now?

[18] The preceding discussion addresses the solutions of: caregiver recruitment and retention and it is key in the standards of care, cost structure and customer value.

Business model development, job and customer satisfaction are also essential in the achieving the mission, vison and values of the organization.

[18] This writer further recommends that solutions value customer expectations that are significant in improving service delivery and job satisfaction for caregivers. While pay and benefits are key in the process, it expands their role and assist the organizational improvement efforts. Although the relationship with the client is paramount, caregivers and staff can serve in a role that assist in creating services that the customer wants e.g. customer jobs. Value proposition design can help "design, test and deliver what customers want."

[19] A. Integrated Suite of Tools the Environmental MAP helps you understand the content which you create.

One map is the first tool. It breaks down the environment into four general categories, (1) market forces, (2) industry forces, 3.) key trends and 4.) macroeconomic forces

Market forces

- Market segments
- Needs and demands
- Market issues
- Switching costs
- Revenue attractiveness

Industry forces

- Supplies
- Stakestoke holders
- Competitors (incumbents)
- New entrants (insurgents)
- Substitute products and services

[20] Solutions cont'd

B. A variety of solutions can be employed to address the critical needs articulated in the thesis. This writer recommends the Baldrige Quality Award process and framework as a beginning journey to performance excellent in healthcare. Organizations are using the VA (Carey Award,) America Healthcare Association, (bronze, silver and gold,) awards, and the coveted Baldrige Award. These awards and the process is encouraged to continue the performance improvement journey.

C. However, to address an immediate need to pursue solutions to current problems. I mentioned the use of the Business Model Generation (Alexander Osterwalder & Yves Pigneur 2010). Utilizing Value Proposition Design. – This approach can create value by those of us who have been displeased with the failure of good ideas and the ability to test and deliver what customers want (Osterwald, Pigneur, Bernada and Smith 2014.)

[21] This model hopes to reach and create value for:

Value propositions that...

- Are based on services that create value for a customer segment (clients and family members.)

Channels Proposition

- Describe how the proposition is communicated to a customer segment.

Customer Relationships

- Outline the type of relationship that is established and maintained with each customer segment, and how they are acquired and retained.

Revenue Streams

- Result from a value proposition successfully offered to a customer segment. It is how an organization captures value with a price customers are willing to pay.

[21] Key Resources

- Are the most important assets required to offer and deliver the previously described elements.

Key Activities

- Are the most important activities an organization needs to perform well.

Key Partnerships

- Shows the networking suppliers and partners that bring in external/extend resources and activities.

Cost Structure

* Describes all costs insured to operate a business model.

Profit

* Is calculated by subtracting the total of all costs in the cost structure from the total of all revenue streams.

[22] The value proposition canvas is divided into two components, value proposition and customer segment.

The value map makes explicit how you believe service will ease pains and create gains. Communicate the map across the organization as a one page document to develop a shared understanding of how you create value. It can be used to track services that actively ease pains and create gains when you test them.

The customer profile helps visualize what matters to customers and their jobs, pains and gains. Communicate the document across the organization to get a shared customer understanding. Use the [23] map to track assumed customer jobs, pains and gains that exist when we talk to real customers. The problem – solutions fit, provides evidence that customers care about their job, pains and gains we want to address with our value proposition product – service market fit. Provides evidence that customers want your value propositions. Business model fit: provides and evidence model for your value proposition is scaleable and profitable. Ibid7.

[24] 10 Characteristics of Great Value Propositions

* Embedded great business models
* Focus jobs, pains and gains that matter to customers.
* Focus on unsatisfied jobs, unresolved pains and unrealized gains.
* Target few jobs, pains and gains, but do so extremely well.

- Go beyond functional jobs and address emotional and social jobs.
- Align with how customers measure success.
- Focus on jobs, pains and gains that a lot of people have or that some will pay a lot of money for.
- **[25]** Differentiate from competition on jobs, pains and gains that customers care about.
- Outperform the competition substantially on at least one dimension.
- Are difficult to copy

CHAPTER 4

Summary

A. Integration of Solutions

The long-term care industry is already established and there are Baldrige role model organizations that are continuously improving. However, to continuously improve the performance excellence process it is important to improve existing value propositions without changing or affecting existing business models. The value proposition design **[26]** Process can improve large existing organizations and or invent new ones. As further recruitment and retention are addressed action research in the form of the value proposition process (VPP) can take place and speed up the process, provide new and improved business models and value propositions. Caregiver recruitment and retention can generate new outcomes for clients now, while policies, procedures and new prototypes come about. Although new to many, the VPP can assist existing organizations **[27]** in improving service delivery to customers and customer segments and generate competitive advantage. As SNF's grapple with the concerns mentioned, caregiver jobs can be expanded and give ownership to the organizational improvement effort and provide further job and customer satisfaction. As market share expands further recruitment and retention efforts can improve and create greater value. "In the End of the Competitive

Advantage," Rita McGrathe talks about "transient advantages" she states companies need to develop the ability to continuously develop the ability [28] to address opportunities rather than search for an sustainable long term advantages.

When building transient advantage, (the ability to constantly improve, improve and deliver value to customers,) it is important to integrate organizational improvement capabilities to leverage opportunity.

At the heart of organization improvement is employee engagement. The Baldrige criteria definition is "the extent of workforce members emotional and intellectual capacity to accomplishing your organizations work, mission and vision. Organizations with high levels of work force engagement are often...environments in which people are motivated to do their upmost to further customer benefit and organizational success." 10.

[29] Again, caregiver recruitment and retention are needed to begin, sustain clinical excellence, standards of care, cost structure and customer value. Business model development, job and customer satisfaction is essential in achieving the mission, vison and values of the organization. Many studies have forced employee engagement noting – non-engaged employees are not self-starters, do not commit to the mission, vision and values and do not delight customers. Kendall and Bodinson 2017, discuss the cost of a disengaged employee they cite "everyone focuses on the cost of employee turnover, and yes those are pretty high. Estimates for recruiting, interviewing, hiring, and training coupled with reduced productivity and lost opportunity costs to replace an employee can be staggering...

[30] They are not going to protect the organizations' resources as if they value their own. They aren't going to look for ways to add value. They aren't going to encourage each other to levels of higher productivity. They aren't going to improve. These types of employees are described as "captives." 11.

Senior leaders must own the employee engagement process. In the book "Teaching the Malcom Baldrige Way" p. 42, states that senior leaders of Poudre Valley Health Services a 2008 Baldrige recipient, indicated that financials are viewed every 30 days while engagement surveys are viewed every 30 months, again senior leaders must "own" the process of caring for employees who are also customers. Span of control of employee to supervision is key in engaging employees and getting their commitment, [31] and compassion to meet customer needs (e.g. customer jobs.) although the Human Capital or of Human Resources department is usually responsible for employee matters, it is the management's role to inculcate participatory leadership, and employee transparency, involvement, particularly with direct care personnel.

When organizations think they are doing well they sometimes have blind spots in other words (they don't know what they don't know). Assessments and checklists can aid in discovering how well they are currently doing with the respect to employee engagement, business model generation around employee engagement (caregiver) and also business model generation as it relates to customers as well as value proposition design.

[32] A key note is that as we look at caregiver recruitment and retention the care givers are also customers of the senior management, and they serve the primary customers and other customer segments. Therefore management's focus must be on the mission, vison and values of the enterprise while simultaneous serving the internal customer employees (i.e. caregivers.) (Baldrige Criteria Category category three.) as far as recruitment goes, a critical need is to get the right people in the right place, therefor employee acquisition is important in employee selection guidelines which are mandated by federal law.

[33] Uniform guidelines and procedures (US EEOE, employee selection.) public law 12.

Qualitative any quantitative data must be taken with account to "get on board" the right people. Objective and subjective criteria must be used to "get the right job." Oftentimes customers in healthcare like and prefer a relationship with their caregivers, not a frequent rotation of caregivers in and out of their lives. Turnover must be limited as much as possible to determine value propositions that lead to customer gains. While recruitment is significant, employee selection must address capacity (i.e. size of the workforce) keeping in mind the critical need of employee engagement.

[33] Also, capability (i.e. workforce skill, knowledge and availability.) one dimension not addressed is that, there is a need to develop skill test(s) for the critical job of caregiver. It has been said that it is easy to get a job as caregiver, however, I maintain that "personality" is critical in this "key position." Critical skill, knowledge and ability alone is not enough to meet the long term care needs of customers in SNF's "personality tests" which are subjective criteria, should be used with objective criteria, to obtain the best and brightest in this important profession. These tests can determine if the employee is suitable for the role of [34] caring for others.

Understanding Customers

Just as important as employee engagement is the need to gain customer insight.
The following six techniques are needed to gain customer insights.

The data detective

- Build on existing (work) research reports and customer data.
- Look at research outside your industry, study analogs, opposites.

Strength – great foundation for further research.
Weakness – statistical data from a different context.

[35] The Journalist

- Talk to customers to gain insight
- Interview may not reveal real world view

Strengths – quick and cheap to get started
Weakness – customers don't always know what they want.

The Anthropologists

- Observe potential customers
- Study jobs customers focus on
- Note pains and gains

Strength – data provides unbiased view, can discover real world weaknesses

Weakness – different to gain insights due to new ideas

These customer insight work with

[36] The Impersonator

- Be your customer
- Spent a day in your customers shoes

Strengths – firsthand experience of jobs, pains and gains.

Weakness – not always representative of real customer.

The Co-creator

- Integrate customers into the process of value creation to learn with them.
- Work with customers to experience new ideas.

Strength – the proximity with customers can gain insight.

Weakness – may not be generalized to all customers and segments.

[37] The Scientist

- Get customers to participate in an experiment (knowing or unknowingly.)
- Work to explore and develop new ideas.

Strength – provides fact based insight or real world behavior.

Weakness – can be hard to apply due to strict policies and guidelines

(Osterwalder et Al 13 Wiley 2014)

[38] These are techniques that work well with employees as costumers too. Valuable insight helps employee customers serve

primary customers. It is important to also help employees understand customer jobs, pains and gains that management is addressing. It also helps that the value position fit the business model.

This process helps align internal and external stake holders.

[39] Based on the 2016 Deloite Mallard Survey "Only 16 percent of millennials see themselves with their current employer a decade from now." Much of the caregiver workforce will be made up of millennials. Distinct value and belief systems separate this cohort from others in the work force. All organizations struggle with retention, however, the best organizations strategically plan for it. Millennials tend to have values that are different from Generation X's, Baby Boomers and traditionalists. They value:

- Employee values programs that satisfy their need for taking care of themselves, in times of physical fitness, health and business.
- May generally value positive indicators or issues they care about (e.g. environment engaging to supervision is key in engaging employees and getting their commitment, compassion to meet customer needs (e.g. customer jobs.) although the Human Capital or Human Resources department is usually responsible for employee matters, it is the management's role to inculocate participatory leadership, and employed involvement particularly with direct care personnel.
- Women's issues and equal opportunity are also important, therefore social responsibly and other corporate programs add value to retention of employees.

When organizations think they are doing well they sometimes have blind spots, in other words they don't know what they don't know. Assessments and checklists can aid in discovering how well they are currently doing with the respect to employee engagement, however business model generation around employee engagement (caregiver) and also business model generation as it relates to customers as well as value proposition design can reduce blind spots.

[40] Millennials value work/life balance (i.e. flexible hours, parental leave, participation in decision making.) the work/ life balance assists employees of the needs fulfill their value proposition. These employees like other employee's value professional development. The belief is that it prepares them in skill set development for future career goals.

[41] Although millennial values are divergent from other workforce cohort groups, they are the "new entrants" to the long term care industry, as services shift along with a shift toward homecare, brand identity, career growth, salary and benefit issues, the need to proactivity address the retention needs of millennials is significant. (Accounting Today) (January 2017. Vol 31 No. 1 January 2017.)

CHAPTER 5

Current Challenges, Policies and Practices

Workforce

Three (3.9) million people receive nursing home assistance. Most participate in Medicare and Medicaid. There are approximately 15,000 plus nursing homes with 1.7 million licensed health care personnel. The onset of Covid-19 pandemic has made both residents and nursing home staff venerable and at risk.

The profile:

- female 90 percent
- minorities 54 percent
- Pacific Islander - 36 percent
- another race/ethnic group 3 percent

Issues

- Recruiting and retaining quality direct care staff
- Turnover rate 51.5 percent

- Staff entered field due to satisfaction from caring for older adults.
- 45 percent of CNA's are very likely to leave their jobs within the year:

(Office of Assistant Secretary for Planning and Evolution "Understanding Direct Care Worker: A snapshot of two America's – https://aspe.hhs.gov/basicreport/understanding-direct-care-workers-snapshot-two-Americas-most-important-jobs).

Wages are an underlying cause of staff shortages, both before and during the Covid-19 pandemic, on average.

CNA's - 14.77 per hour

Nursing Assistants - 14.25 per hour

RN's - 33.53 per hour, 11 percent than the industry average.

Although, wages have increased marginally, they have not kept with infraction.

Key facts

- Approximately 15,600 nursing homes operate across the nation.
- 69% of nursing homes have for profit ownership, 24% are nonprofit and 7% are government owned/other
- 62% of nursing home residents have Medicaid as their primary payer.
- 6% of nursing homes have 0-25 occupants
- 64% have 26-100 occupants,
- 30% have 100+ occupants

Source: https://www.cdc.gov/nchs/data/series/SRO3-43-508.pdf.

Staffing was continued to be cursive and since the 1987 Nursing Home Reformat, the staffing levels have not been adjusted in over 30 years, with increased capacity of baby boomers. Medicare patients receive approximately $500 per day, needing post-acute skilled care, compared to Medicaid residents who receive lower compensation.

On March 27, 2020, 100 billion in Provider relief funds supported hospitals, on April 24, 2020, Skill Nursing Facilities (SNFs) received 4.9 billion received federal stimulus on May 22, 2020; as a release of 5 billion from the Provider Relief Fund for SNFs.

Practices

While nursing homes are designed for short and long term care for chronic conditions and disabilities, a paucity of understanding related to transmission of Covid-19 infection prevention means, they were not positioned to address surge in Covid-19 infections. Staff shortages further impact services to residents. A lack of dedicated in-room sinks which impact the problem due to a lack of residents that receive direct personal care, makes it difficult to address infection control - prevention. "Few if any, nursing homes have rooms designed for isolation with negative air flow or allow for respiratory isolation in the event of pathogens such as Covid-19." https://aspe/hhs.gov/basic-report/Covid-19-intensifies-nursing-home-workforce-challenges.p.9

Summary of Key Findings

- Staffing shortages and attrition have further strained nursing homes during the pandemic. In response some nurses and CNAs staff are leaving the sector during this critical time when there is an increased demand.
- To mitigate the impact of Covid-19 on staffing levels, nursing homes are developing new recruitment infrastructure, credentialing requirements and deploy nontraditional staff for surge support.
- To retain nursing home staff and other frontline healthcare workers Federal State, and local governments should provide benefits such as childcare, housing transportation assistance and food supports.

- The lack of a unified testing strategy, test kits, and an approach to covering the cost of testing reportedly delayed understanding about the risk of Covid-19 transmission.
- To prevent and control Covid-19 infections among nursing home staff and residents, federal and state governments, instituted non-leave policies, and monitored staff for illness. (IBID)

Conclusion

Caregiver recruitment and retention must sustain standards of care, cost structure and customer value. Business model development, jobs and customer satisfaction are essential.

Lastly, the position of this writer in view of a recent newspaper article, US nursing home staffing falls as patients seek help. St. Louis Post Dispatch 10.08.2021 Friday am, the nursing home crisis in getting worse. "One in three nursing homes has fewer nurses and aides than before the Covid-19 pandemic highlighted the truth of a profit driven industry with too few caring for the society's most vulnerable". "In a June survey, the American Health Care Association (AHCA) found nursing homes were losing revenue due to fewer patients coming from hospitals, and nearly half of nursing homes and assisted living facilities had made cuts". I maintain caregivers need and deserve higher pay, increased benefits and improved federal, state and local policy initiatives to truly care for others. Truly society's most vulnerable deserve better.

References

1. A Perfect Stows: High Turnover Coupled with Increasing Demand for LTC Workers. March 19, 2015 Freve, Flesche Retention in Long-Term Care Professionals: Assessing the Challenges. Janice Heineman, PhD IFAS, AAHSA

2. IFAS (Institute for the Future of Aging Services) AAHSA Talent Cabinet January 2010 31 American Association of Homes and Services for Aging (AAHSA)

3. Singh, DA. & Schwab, R.C. (1998) Retention of Administration in Nursing homes: What can management do? The Gerontologist, 40 (3):310-319

4. Castle N.G. & Engberg J (2006) Organizational Characteristic associated with staff turnover in nursing homes. The Gerontologist 46 (1):62-73???.

5. Whitaker T. Weisminer, T. and Clark, E (2006).
Assuring the sufficiency of a frontline workforce: A national study of licensed social workers.
Special report: Social work services for older adults.
Washington, D.C. National association of social workers (NASW)

6. Institute for the Future of Aging Services (IFAS). The long-term care work force: Can the crisis be fixed? January 2007.

7. Osterwalder, A., Pigneur, Y., Bernarda, G., Smith, A., "Value Proposition Design"
   2014 Wiley

8. Osterwalder, A. Pigneur, Y. Business Model Generation – 2010 Wiley

9. McGrath, Rita "The End of Harvard Business Competitive Advantage" 2013 review

10. The Malcolm Baldrige. National Quality Improvement of 1987, Public Law 100-107 Act. http://www.nist.gov/blardige/about/improvement

11. Leading the Malcolm Baldrige Way. Kay Kendall, Glenn Bodinson, Mcgraw - McGraw – Hill 2017

12. Albert, Link and John T. Scott, Economic Evaluation of the Baldrige Performance Excellance
    Program, December 2011 http://nist.gov

13. Uniform Guidelines on Employee Selection Procedures
    1978   www.eeoc.gov
           www.opm.gov
           www.dol.gov
    2019   uniform guidelines.gov

14. Tour, Rogowski Accounting Today, January 2017. Vol 1 No 1